DEDICATION
To all my beautiful readers

Disclaimer

DEFINING ADDICTION. AM I AN ALCOHOLIC? 7

   HOW TO KNOW WHEN YOU DRINK EXCESSIVELY? 9
   TYPICAL SIGNS OF ALCOHOLISM...9

UNDERSTANDING WHY YOU DRINK 11

   I ONLY DRINK TO BE SOCIABLE...11
   DRINKING MAKES ME HAPPY 13
   ALCOHOL GIVES ME COURAGE 15
   IT'S GENETIC...18
   IT'S CULTURAL. I NEED TO DRINK TO FIT IN...21
   BOREDOM...24
   STRESS 26
   IT HELPS ME RELAX...30
   UNDER THE INFLUENCE 33
   IT'S A HABIT..36

REINFORCEMENT: THE DRIVER OF CHANGE..38

IS ALCOHOL VITAL TO SOCIAL LIFE? 41

IS IT A HABIT? 44

DIFFERENT SOLUTIONS 46

WHO AM I AFFECTING?..49

STAYING AWAY FROM THE FIRST DRINK 51

THE MYTH OF THE ADDICTIVE PERSONALITY 53

THOSE LUCKY NORMAL DRINKERS 57

HOW TO MAKE IT EASY TO QUIT 59

THE FINAL DRINK 62

CAN'T SEEM TO QUIT DRINKING?..64

   YOUR SYSTEM DEMANDS IT 64
   LACK OF WILL POWER..65
   LACK OF COUNSELING...65
   NOT READY TO QUIT 66

13 AMAZING REASONS TO STOP DRINKING 67

START WITH 15-DAYS OF SOBRIETY 70

TAKE ONE DAY AT A TIME 70

   DAY 1 70
   DAY 2 71
   DAY 3 71
   DAY 4 72
   DAY 5 72
   DAY 6 73
   DAY 7 73
   DAY 8 74
   DAY 9 74
   DAY 10 75
   DAY 11 75
   DAY 12 76
   DAY 13 76
   DAY 14 77
   DAY 15 77

WHAT IF I TRIP? 79

   SOBRIETY TIMELINE 81

DEALING WITH GUILT 83

LIFE AFTER ADDICTION 87

Defining addiction. Am I an alcoholic?

First, let's try to define the alcoholic addiction. Alcoholism is when person is dependent on alcohol, the situation when the individual has a physical or psychological need to drink alcohol. Alcohol abuse refers to a certain pattern of behavior (this refers to situations when a person drinks too much in a situation that carries certain negative consequences).

How to know if you are an alcoholic? Maybe you don't fit the stereotypes, you don't steal the money to drink, and you have home, family, friends and job. There are many different forms of alcoholism, so yours may be atypical.

You are probably wondering when a drink or two with friends converts to a problem. I would start with casual drinking. It's quite common, especially nowadays, to have a couple of drinks with friends, or with dinner or maybe at some party. Unless you don't have some restrictions because of your health or maybe religion this is all right. The problems can begin if you start abusing alcohol.

It's quite usual that people think that the terms "alcoholism" and "alcohol abuse" is the same thing. Well, they're not. Alcoholism is an alcohol addiction or dependence, where the individual has some physical or psychological need to drink alcohol. Alcohol abuse is a pattern of behavior (when a person drinks in spite of the negative consequences).

For people younger than 65 heavy drinking means to have more than 14 drinks in one week or four or more in one day. For people older than 65, it means more than seven drinks in one week or three drinks a day.

If a person drinks more than this (in other words a large amount of alcohol such as five or more drinks in two hours) he is a binge drinker. If we refer to women this is for four or more drinks in one occasion.

Typical signs of alcoholism

If heavy or binge drinking happens once in a blue moon than it's not such a big problem for you. But if this becomes more often, pay attention to some signs and use them as a warning.

Neglecting responsibilities is maybe the first sign. If you start with low performance at work or at school, if you do not pay attention to your kids, you forget to pick them up or some of their daily routine or maybe you start avoiding meetings because you're drunk or hung over this is a sign for you to immediately stop.

Putting yours or other people's lives in danger and driving drunk (or in a worst scenario start mixing medications with alcohol) is definitely a sign that something is not right.

It became normal in modern American culture to have a drink after a long day at work or after an argument with someone you love. Once or twice it won't be a problem but this can turn into a need.

If you drink in spite of the fact that this causes problems in your relationship or family, if you notice that everyone criticize you because of alcohol, be aware that you've got serious problem.

Understanding why you drink

Many people think that drinking alcohol is nothing more than a nice way to relax. People, who are alcohol addicted, drink to excess. They lose the fact that they harm not only themselves but others as well. I'll present you some of the commonest reasons for drinking alcohol.

I only drink to be sociable

A person who occasionally takes a couple of drinks is, we could say, "a casual drinker". This means approximately one or two glasses of wine with dinner after a hard working day or a few bears (of course occasionally, not all the time).

Someone who drinks (again occasionally) with friends (at friend's home, in a bar, at the party), is "a social drinker". Just to repeat, this is when things can get messy. Why? It's a thin line between a social drinker and addicted person. The difference is whether you are going to be a casual drinker who has a drink or two with his or her friends, or to become too much intoxicated. The amount of the alcohol you take in during a day is very important.

If your only reason to drink is to be sociable my opinion is that you shouldn't do that. If you drink to please your friends, make a polite excuse and say no. If, on the other hand, you enjoy having a drink or two with them, it's ok. It's not uncommon to see people who once hated alcohol become addicted. So, if you need a drink or two, take it and enjoy. If you only drink to be accepted by others, don't drink. There are many other ways to be accepted and enjoy time with your friends that don't include alcohol. It doesn't mean that you are sociable if you drink alcohol.

Alcohol does wonders for the soul. It can help you to cool off and relax. It can also reduce the stress levels. If you are worried or concerned, it can help you relax and have fun. But, if you consume too much alcohol, it may have negative effect on your body and health.

Scientist organized some researches recently to test whether or not happiness levels are directly connected with drinking alcohol. With these information set they uncovered that drinking alcohol increases the level of happiness. Next, they wanted to check if there are some specific activities that cause this condition. They discovered that drinking makes fun activities just a little more enjoyable but it really eases doing something you don't want or is boring to you.

But, the scientists also determined that drinking increases levels of happiness for a short period of time. So, it doesn't have long lasting effect. And one more thing, if drinkers start relying on alcohol too much to increase their happiness eventually it will make them less happy. To conclude, drinking can make you happier but it won't last long. It is fun and can make you stressed out. But, be careful because there is a great possibility that you get addicted rather than happy. Choose some other things like family and friends to make you happy, not alcohol.

It is quite common for a person to take a drink before a certain stressful moment. This implies to situations such as asking someone to go out with you or when preparing for an important meeting or presentation.

People usually believe that alcohol makes them braver. Alcohol relaxes our muscles. It makes us lose control eventually. This happens even if we are not aware of it. We feel stressed out, less nervous. These facts enable us to feel more self-confident. On the one hand, this makes us believe we are braver; we feel freer than in situations in which we are sober. On the other hand, this can cause a problem. Why? When we are under the influence of alcohol we sometimes can't control our emotions. This is not a normal state of our mind. We may express our emotions in an exaggerated   way.

We often think this is courage. What alcohol actually does to us is that it lowers inhibitions. That can make us behave the way we normally wouldn't. I have to admit that there are certain situations in which this is good and will result positively. But there are many more situations in which we can do or say something bad rather than good. Some of the commonest examples of bad behavior under the influence of alcohol are aggression and violence. To make this worse we could do something like this in front of people we normally wouldn't. We have to accept and first of all to understand that alcohol doesn't give us courage or self- confidence. It just lowers the blocks in our brain.

Let's see how alcohol affects us. First of all, it has numerous neurological effects, such as memory loss, slowed reflexes, it can make us feel sleepy, and many other things that aren't good for us, like lowered inhibitions. As previously mentioned, lowered inhibitions can make us do or say something we'll regret later.

If we discuss an actual courage or boost in confidence, we can't say there are many evidence to support this theory from neurological point of view. However, people will tell you that they feel braver or more self-confident while being influenced by the alcohol. How? Well, if you believe that alcohol makes you into a better or prettier person than you probably won't need more than one beer to make you do something brave, or something really stupid.

In some situations the courage that alcohol provides, or more exactly the courage that you think alcohol provides, really comes in handy (important business meeting, a date with someone you really like-when the challenge is too big and the pressure is very high). The problem arises if you need a drink to get out because you need to take the garbage out or when you want to call your mother, father, etc. (so, some ordinary stuff).

It's really important not to cross the line. This means you should be careful and have some limits in behavior. Don't just say what's on your mind. Unfortunately, people often can't control themselves when they are drunk. The biggest problem is when you are rude. This leads to damage and, maybe a missing tooth.

Always have in mind that drunken people look dangerous to others. They are not anyone's top choice, especially if they cause problems. You don't need alcohol to be brave and make decision. Have in mind that you can stand up for yourself or ask someone out without alcohol. If you, on the other hand need it badly, make sure that you don't take too much alcohol and stay cool.

Dithering about whether alcohol use disorder runs in a family or not is very common. Among scientists it's not unusual to hear about an "alcoholism gene." According to them, genetics has certain influence, but the story isn't so simple.

What does the science say? Studies show that genes play roll and are responsible for about half of the risk for this gene. But, genes cannot determine if someone will develop an alcoholism gene. There are many other factors along with genes that influence the risk.

What's the situation with genes? Well, there are some genes that increase a risk, as well as those that decrease the risk. This is caused directly or indirectly. Some people have bigger chances to develop addiction than others but this doesn't have to mean that they will. In some cases things can be easier for those who are aware of the presence of this gene because they are alerted in advance and can be cautious.

Different factors can change the expression of this gene. This is the field of epigenetics. Scientists are trying to explore this field as much as possible. Epigenetics is a branch of genetics that deals with the factors that turn genes on and off. The development of this branch is very important because it can give us useful information about things we should avoid if we don't want to activate certain genes (not only related to alcoholism but as well other diseases).

Many scientific studies have shown that genetic factors influence alcoholism. These studies show that kids of alcoholics are four times more likely than others to develop alcohol problems. It's a fact that children of alcoholics also have a higher risk for many emotional and problems with behavior. But I have to point out that this is not crucial. It's not necessarily for children of alcoholics to become alcoholics as well. An alcoholic parent isn't the determiner of an alcoholic child. In fact, more than a half of children of alcoholics don't become alcoholics. There are many other factors that form an alcoholic.

Different aspects of life influence and increase the risk for alcoholism. The way parents act and treat each other and the children also influences on children's growing up. There are some situations in family that will increase the risk:

If a parent is depressed
If a parent has some other psychological problems
If a parent abuses drugs and alcohol
If there is a history of violent behavior in the family.

The good side is that most children of alcoholics (even from the most troubled families) don't have drinking problems. A family history of alcoholism and bad behavioral and communicational skills do not guarantee that a child will become an alcoholic or a bad person. Even though the risk is high it doesn't have to happen.

If you know that you come from such a family avoid underage drinking. First, it's illegal. Second, research shows that the risk is higher for those who start drinking at an early age. Then, don't drink too much when you grow up. This doesn't only refer to people from problematic families but others as well. So, no more than a drink a day for women, and two drinks a day for men. There are some people who shouldn't drink at all (pregnant or women who are trying to become pregnant, drivers, recovering alcoholics, people who take certain medications, people with certain medical conditions).

If you notice any kind of problems you should talk to a health care professional and discuss your problems with a doctor. He or she can help you by recommending groups or organizations that work with people with alcoholic problems and can help you avoid them. If you have already begun to drink, a professional can help you deal with it. Don't make any excuses if you need any kind of help because disposing can destroy your life.

There are many different social and cultural roles of alcohol. Different researches have shown that these roles of alcohol can have important impact on drinking culture. This is global, not related to a particular country or culture.

This issue is closely connected with politics and it is essential for political leaders and those who deal with legislation on alcohol to clearly understand the socio-cultural functions of drinking and how they influence people's lives.

Alcohol has a certain symbolic role. It is obvious that in all cultures where more than one type of alcoholic beverage is available, they are categorized according to their social meaning. This classification defines the social world. Every drink is loaded with symbolic meaning, every drink carries a message. Alcohol has a very powerful role in cultural systems (manipulation, description, construction of those systems). Choice of a drink is rarely a matter of personal taste. It's commonly dictated.

Beverages are usually situation definers. You wonder how? Well, in many cultures (especially Western) drinks define the nature of the occasion. Champagne is synonym for celebration. This is so deep into culture that any time we see someone drinking champagne we will wonder what he or she celebrates. Schnapps, for example, is reserved for intimate gatherings. Wine is considered an appropriate accompaniment to a meal. Different types of wine are considered appropriate for celebrations, while beer is the most appropriate drink for informal, relaxing situations. In some cultures (such as French) there is a determined order we should respect. The aperitif is drunk before the meal; white wine goes before red wine or brandy. There are different rules in different cultures and if you refuse to follow them it may be offensive for the host.

Alcohol is status indicator. It indicates social status. Imported drinks have a higher status than the local ones. Preference for expensive and imported drinks is more a kind of an aspiration than it actually shows social status. Alcoholic beverage can also show membership, generation, special group people belong to, nation, beliefs, attitude, political status, etc. We have situations of certain drinks becoming symbols of national identity (tequila-Mexico, Guinness-Ireland, ouzo-Greece).

The usage of different beverages can also symbolize the age. Younger generations are opened for new choices while the older people follow tradition. Therefore, we can say that alcohol is also gender differentiator. Almost all societies and cultures make distinction between masculine and feminine drinks as well.

Alcohol has a big cultural role but there isn't any significant cross-cultural study of this phenomenon, only occasional two-country comparison.

There is one thing we should especially pay attention to. It seems that adopting foreign drinks also involves adopting drinking patterns of foreign cultures and countries.

Putting all pieces together we can conclude that what all cultures have in common is that they nurse drinking alcohol as an important part of celebrations and as an important social act. I don't think this is extremely bad, I only advice drinking moderately.

You probably ask yourself what does boredom has to do with alcohol and alcoholism. Unfortunately, these two are closely connected. The fact is that boredom is often a reason why someone experiments with alcohol or some other substance in a first place. It is also quite common that people who are treated from alcoholism use boredom as an excuse to keep coming back to alcohol. There is a constant feeling of fear that life without alcohol will be boring.

Boredom is a condition or, someone would say a feeling that, sooner or later, we all experience. This happens when we don't have anything to do or there is lack of interest for everything around us. There are different types of boredom such as: when there is nothing we want to do, when there is something we aren't allowed to do and when we can't stay focused on anything (we lose interest easily).

Boredom is a part of life. As mentioned we all experience it eventually. The only trouble is that it can be very dangerous. It may seem funny but it's a very common reason for addiction of any kind. Chronic boredom is very dangerous because it can cause different addictions, among others alcoholism.

Recent survey has shown that about thirty percent of teenagers turn to alcohol in the state of boredom. People commonly turn to alcohol since they've got nothing else to do. Repeating this leads to addiction.

This is extremely dangerous for people who are in recovery. I use the word extremely because alcohol destroys people's lives as well as homes and families and it's important to point that out. These people are scared that they won't have anything else to because the one thing they really enjoy is alcohol. For some people the state of boredom is rather trivial while for other represents a huge problem. It's highly important for these people to get involved in different activities or to find new hobbies. You wouldn't believe how big effort escaping boredom requires.

The boredom is often an excuse for relapses to return to alcohol. They have to find a meaning or a purpose, especially in first days of their recover, or they will come back to alcohol.

The best thing is to avoid boredom. You have to be in charge, you must take control of your life. There isn't a better way to avoid boredom and alcohol abuse than this. You can try finding a new hobby or plan things ahead. Escaping the routine is one more way. Push yourself; find new adventures or maybe some new friends. Find anything that will keep you away from boredom.

We live very stressfully today. A modern man is exposed to many stressful situations every day. Many studies show that people start drinking in order to cope with modern life. This implies economic situation, job problems, marital problems, and many others. Today's way of life and its speed can be unbearable. While a drink after hard day at work and over dinner from time to time is all right, habitual repeating of this can lead to excess.

The worst is prolonged stress. This is independent on whether a person comes from a family with history of alcoholism or not. Different levels of stress cause different quantity and frequency of alcohol consumption. If there is no support through other alternatives or social-BOM, there is an alcoholic in the announcement.

And, if a person believes that alcohol helps to reduce the stress in his or her life, alcohol is most likely to always be used as a response to stress.

It's not easy to establish a clear connection between stress, drinking and alcoholism among people. Why? It's hard to make clear connections because it appears that what is stressful for one person is not necessarily stressful for another. And there are many other factors that also need to be included in order to determine these connections.

Nowadays, there are many types of stress. They are related with different part of people's lives and with different situations. How one will deal with stress depends on many factors such as environment, support, how he or she copes with stressful situations and many others. We've already mentioned that there are many types of stress. But, there is one specific type of stress today that more and more people have to deal with. That is the stresses associated with military service. People who come back from war zones or those who, from some reason, leave the active duty are exposed to specific type of stress. The transformation of life can be very hard and these people very often start consuming alcohol just to go throughout a day. Not rarely, they become alcoholics. Some other situations that not small number of people will find stressful are: a new job, a death of someone close (friends, family), moving, getting married or divorced, to break up, etc. All these situations may result in numerous changes in us and cause stress. One way that people choose to deal with it is turning to alcohol. Drinking alcohol may lead to relaxation and reducing stress. The real problems appear, when stress is ongoing and people continue dealing with it by drinking.

The situation may be reversed. Someone who has quite normal life without too much stress may start drinking (boredom, culture, etc.-we've mentioned these causes earlier). This can cause their lives tear apart. Alcoholics often lose their jobs, friends, family, get divorced. They simply lose everything and often continue to drink not realizing that alcohol actually caused all of their problems.

The ability to deal with stress is called resilience. That is actually the reflection of how well someone is able to deal with stressful situations.

Once we feel stressed our body responds quickly, shifting normal metabolic processes into high ones. To make this quick response possible, the body releases adrenalin. Our system prepares the body either to fight the stress or to escape it.

The hormone called cortisol has a key role in our body's response to stress. It increases our energy by increasing blood sugar levels and nutrient supplies to the muscles. This is how our organism prepares our body to respond efficiently and quickly.

We are resilient when we are able to respond quickly to stress. However, not every organism will react in a right way and many factors will determine the respond (personality, lifestyle, immune system, environmental factors, etc.). It's important to focus on positive things, stay optimistic, and solve problems. This is the best way to deal with stress.

The link between the stress and alcohol abuse always existed. But, it has become especially relevant over the last few decades because of the increased abuse of alcohol. Alcohol became one of the most commonly used means to free from stress.

Alcohol imitates the action of a neuro-inhibitor and slows down the release of an excitatory neurotransmitter. This causes our experience of reality seem slower and we start feeling relaxed. This can be good and useful in some situations because it will make us feel more comfortable.

Drinking alcohol to relax is a common appearance. People find that alcohol helps them lose stress. Alcohol slows down brain activity and in a certain way masks feelings of stress, and anxiety or pressure. At the same time improves our mood.

You must remember next- you should never use alcohol as a solution. Very often people drink after a fight or quarrel or when they are under pressure. People also drink to escape problems, disappointment, boredom or to fit in. This is wrong. This can easily convert to alcohol abuse.

It's risky to drink alcohol to relax. Why? It can increase person's chances of building a dependence on alcohol and this leads to addiction. People sometimes don't believe that occasional drinking creates the risk of alcoholism. Drinking alcohol to relax is a kind of defensive mechanism. The danger this mechanism carries is that, in most cases, people begin relying on alcohol whenever they face problems. Every new stressful situation and problem will lead to a new drink and soon we'll need a drink whenever we want to relax.

You must learn how to relax without alcohol. Always have in mind that this is just a partial solution. It won't help you in the long run. Learning how to relax in stressful situations without alcohol is extremely important.

At first, it looks like drinking relaxes us. We feel stressed-out and calm. We feel less shy and generally relaxed. The effect that alcohol has on our brain is similar to those medications against antianxiety have. So, this is not a solution. As I've already mentioned, it's ok to have a drink or two if you are nervous before a date or an important meeting in your company or after a hard day of work. Alcohol will slow down your brain functions and you'll feel relaxed. Occasionally, this is not a problem. But if you start drinking every time you feel anxious or nervous you can easily become addicted. The feeling of relaxation is short. Eventually, you'll have to come back to the real world. Alcohol shouldn't be the answer to your problems. It's important to point out that there are many other ways to lose stress and relax. You can start practicing in a gym, or go jogging. You can read, hang out with your friends. Alcohol is not the answer to your problems. Bread in, bread out and find another solution.

Drinking alcohol is widespread. People start drinking alcohol under different influences and under different ages.

Younger people usually drink more frequently than the elderly (this is not always the case but it's more common). This happens especially if they live in a family where a family member drinks, and also, if they aren't under the supervision of parents or have easy access to alcohol.

Friends play a critical role in this while family has a strong influence. Parents have a strong influence on their child's behavior. This means that parents have to follow their children's behavior from the time they first try alcohol. This also refers to number of times they (the children) go out, where they go, who they go with, are there any other changes in their behavior, etc. It's important that parents have things under control but to avoid choking their children because this might have the opposite effect.

Increasing alcohol consumption among young people, especially younger than 18 is worried. It is still not totally clear which factors have the most influence. There are some factors that appear to be the most common: family, friends, media and celebrity.

So, we saw that alcohol consumption can be caused by different influences. When it comes to young people the strongest factor are friends who drink alcohol. If a child has friends who often drink he or she will probably start drinking. This is inevitable but don't freak out, there is always something you can do. A parent can explain to his child what bad influence alcohol has on his or her organism, how he or she can become addicted. A parent can also show a video or something similar to his or her child in order to sketch this.

Family influence is also a very strong. Family drinking habits are very important. If a child comes from a family with history of alcohol abuse it is highly possible (not always) to start drinking. It's crucial for a child to grow in a healthy and supportive family. Supervision is also important. A parent has to know about his children's movements, where does a child spend time, how and who with.

Alarm doesn't turn on when a person drinks occasionally. It turns on when a person starts drinking excessively. There are different factors here as well. The drinking level of person's friends can determine that person's drinking level. Alcohol is very available nowadays and this is the most dangerous. Every person older than 18 can buy it. So if a child or young adult has someone who is older and can buy alcohol among his or her friends a parent should really pay attention.

Other important influencers (besides friends and family) are celebrities. Their behavior influences young people attitude toward many things a lot and alcohol and drinking is no exception.

When it comes to bad influences there is nothing much we can do. We can provide a healthy, supportive and strong family. We can talk to our children and try explaining what is so bad in alcohol, especially in excessive drinking. It is eventually up to a person to decide what's good and what's bad.

Let's see what a habit is. Everything you are now is the sum of your habits. Whether you are over overweight, or you can't maintain relationships, or you are successful, loved among people-it's dependent on your habits. Our habits define almost everything we are and we do. A habit is a regular practice. It's hard to give up habits. Everything we do over and over again a long period of time is a habit. The longer we repeat something we do the harder it is to stop it. It's the same with alcohol. This makes things pretty hard. It's not easy to break habits. It may sometimes take years to lose a certain habit. Image how hard can that be when drinking is one of your habits. First, you have to be persistent. You need to make a firm decision that you don't want to repeat the habit of drinking. Search out for a trigger (it can be an action or an exact situation when you feel like you need a drink) and remove it. Change the habit. For example, if you always need a drink before an important business meeting or a project, tell yourself (without giving up) that you simply can do that without alcohol. Maybe it won't work first or second time, or for a month or two but eventually it has to and it will. Plan how to do this. Maybe you will (in this example) go jogging before the meeting, or you'll call someone you trust to talk to (telling him or her about the problem) or any other way that's convenient for you. Then, don't set the time-don't pressure yourself too much. As I said habits are hard to be broken, so take your time. Remember "Still waters run deep". Once you succeed, enjoy.

Reinforcement: the driver of change

Reinforcement is a term used in a process of increasing frequency of behavior that is desirable. In this process that desirable behavior is aided by reward. This means that someone is rewarded if he or she shows that desirable behavior but as well punished (in a certain way) for undesired behavior. From this point of view we've got positive and negative reinforcement. Different incentive programs are type of a reward. Reinforcement is a system or a process which can be used for many different things and alcohol rehab is one of them.

If reinforcement is a process of initiation, positive reinforcement is giving a reward while negative reinforcement is the removal of an undesired condition.

This is very useful thing when it comes to different forms of addictive behavior. It's a good tool that can be used to help people who created any form of addiction.

Reinforcement is used to install a certain type of behavior and to uninstall the other. This process **is not** as simple as it seems. It's not rare that it is misunderstood. This is not simply a system of reward or punishment. It is psychological process that is meant to cause repetition of certain behaviors. When it comes to alcohol abuse, this can be very helpful. Why? Well, because reinforcement can create desirable behavior.

Reinforcement is an action that causes a repetition of some behavior more frequently. Positive reinforcement is, as we've already mentioned, when the subject receives a reward for good behavior. This reward should cause that behavior to be repeated. Negative reinforcement also causes a repetition, but here, the action causes a bad feeling or situation to go away.

For people with alcohol abuse problems, rewards of abuse were probably learned long ago (consuming alcohol brings a feeling of pleasure). It's dangerous when a good feeling starts to fade because a person will turn to alcohol again. This is negative reinforcement. The trouble with alcohol is that it provides a relief and a sort of escape from troubles and stress (this causes a constant come-back to alcohol even though it's role of de-stressor doesn't last).

There are different treatment options for applying negative and positive reinforcements in alcohol abuse cases. One way is to try eliminating the stressful situation that causes alcohol consumption. Another way is to allow the patient to meet the stressor face to face and change the habit by finding another way to deal with the problem or situation. Positive and negative reinforcements can be successful treatment in alcohol abuse cases, especially if the problem is accompanied by depression or anxiety.

Is alcohol vital to social life?

Before we even tried alcohol we didn't need it to enjoy, spend time with friends and family. We played with other kids; we listened to music, everything without alcohol. Then, as we grew older, you noticed that everyone around us drinking in different social situations. In fact, I believe that we have never seen such situations without alcohol. So, what happened? We assumed alcohol is a key ingredient for a good party.

First, we begin to drink socially. Since alcohol is a part of almost every social event, soon the only way we could socialize was with alcohol. With time we developed a small dependence (small because if there was no alcohol available it was still ok). But, soon we didn't have as much fun as when we drank. Conclusion- alcohol is a key to social life. We must point out one thing- there is no such thing as clear drinking. In many occasions, alcohol can turn a great party into a nightmare (weddings for example).

As human beings, we are predicted to commute with others. But we are also rational and for that reason we should be aware of what's good and what's bad for us. Social activities can play an important role in preventing addiction. Spend time doing social activities. Alcohol won't let this happen. From the experience of people who I personally know and that were addicted, alcohol brings loneliness. People who are alcohol addicts lose connection with other people. They keep many secrets and consider that alcohol is better than people. They say it is hard to admit this but it's true. Alcohol doesn't make things nice, friends do (and everything they are and do).

We've already talked about how alcohol influences our brain and what effect it has. For a certain period of time it makes us feel better, but not for long. Then it starts destroying. It can take ten days to alcohol fully leave our system, and during that time we simply need a drink. People don't even notice this. We had fun and now we believe that alcohol helps us have fun. Eventually, we really believe this and we start thinking that there is no fun without alcohol. If we skip a drink, we feel bad. In all this we forget to look around and see that there are so many people out there who don't drink and yet have fun. Sooner then we realize, we become slaves of alcohol. Our social events become monotonous and boring and sometimes, we can't even remember where we were and what happened.

People who stopped drinking will tell you that now (when they don't drink anymore) have much more fun than they did before. They are now able to actually enjoy social events, talk to people, hang out, and remember things. Neither one of them lost anything but alcohol, but they gained a lot.

Remember that it's not social to get drunk and have a fight, or to throw up and lose consciousness. Social is to remember things you did with your friends and family, where you have been, who with, who won the game, etc. And next time when someone offers you a drink, think twice whether you really need that to have fun.

Is it a habit?

Is alcoholism a disease or a habit? Let's see. You'll find that many alcoholics give so many excuses when it comes to explaining their situation. They usually want to make things sound confusing. Most of them will tell you that you don't understand. This way they give themselves excuse for drinking and at the same time they don't take responsibility for their actions.

You will hear many excuses from addicted alcoholics. They will try to explain that for example, it's a habit they've inherited from their parent or parents who also had the habit of drinking every day. They expect excuses to make their situation more understandable (for them alcoholism runs in the family, and there's nothing they can do about it).

Alcoholism usually starts as a habit and we've already talked about that in this book. You start with your friends when you first start going out. It continues as a solution in some complicated or stressful situations like a relief. This is when you probably have a drink or two. This won't arise into bigger problem if you know how to stop. But if you start drinking every time you feel stressed and see no other way to deal with problems, the trouble is on its way.

But if you tell an alcoholic that he suffers from a disease, there is a big possibility that you'll give him one more excuse. That's what actually makes things so hard. He or she might simply accept the excuse of illness like "I'm sick, there is nothing I can do".

Honestly, we shouldn't see alcoholism as a disease because that can give people an easy way out. This is their way to hide behind an excuse and avoid solutions. We should see alcoholism as something that can be beaten if we are committed enough to change our habits.

First and most important you must have a personal reason and a desire to fight back. You have to find a reason to do so. The reasons will differ among different people, but any reason that will keep you away from drinking is a good reason (a boyfriend/a girlfriend, family, job, etc.). It has to be something worth fighting for.

The bottom line is that alcoholism addiction is not a disease (it shouldn't be seen as a disease), it's just a bad habit. And, like other bad habits we have, we can change this. It's just a matter of our wish to change things. We have to be devoted and do it day by day. If we are persistent enough, we'll eventually lose this bad habit.

Different solutions

Alcoholism is one of the most common forms of substance abuse in many countries. The approach to dealing with alcohol addiction is highly important. It's necessary to find the right approaches if we want to help people to handle this problem in a right way and forever. Short term programs focus on abstinence but this, almost always gives short-term results. Solving problems with alcoholism requires thorough approach and above all time and support. Knowing all the facts is a first step. It's important to know the facts about why someone started drinking in a first place. We must be armed with the facts if we want to help. Alcohol is a like a drug used against depression. The effect of alcohol depends on how much someone drinks. After the first drink, a person receives a stimulant effect. That person starts feeling more calm and sees alcohol as a solution. If this turns into a habit this person might lose control. The judgment is damaged in a way. Alcohol is available in many forms, under different names but its effect is the same.

A group that needs the solutions most is teenagers. Their age is very sensitive, especially the part when they enter puberty. At this age they are very sensitive. The other sensitive group is young adults. They often drink several drinks in a short period of time (especially when they go out with their friends). The effect of alcohol is delayed (our body is trying to cope with it). The worst consequence of this is death. How? Because of this postponed effect, a person can drink so much; at levels so toxic for him or her to survive (there is a big possibility that he or she won't even notice this).

Before you start providing help you need to make sure that a person is actually an alcoholic. There are many signs of alcoholism and I will try to show you the most important. These signs can show you whether to react or not. One of them is a huge desire for drinking (the alcoholic feels compulsion). We can add loss of control (drinking without limits). And of course, if you notice that someone can't function without alcohol, you can be sure that he is an alcoholic.

Alcoholism is a huge problem, not only for alcoholic but his environment as well.

Let's see what some solutions are. The best way is when an alcoholic admits that he's got problems and makes a decision to solve these problems. In this case he will ask for help, from his or her friends or family, or from a person qualified. The support is necessary because this is not an easy trip. Addiction doesn't stop after the body is free from the immediate impact of alcohol. For heavy drinkers medical detoxification is necessary. Detoxification is a first step but not the last. It's important to find the cause. It can be hard for an alcoholic to tell why he started drinking in a first place and this is where supporting groups can help. It's sometimes easier to tell your problem to a stranger (especially when that person has or had similar problem) than to a close person. The cause must be either solved or accepted. Alcoholic needs to heal his mind not only body

Next step is making yourself busy. Go to the gym, enroll some new course, or find an extra job. Keep yourself busy and surrounded by people you care about. There are also different exercises and nutrition programs that can help. There are many ways, you just have to decide and start.

Who am I affecting?

Alcoholics affect everyone, their family, friends, partners, colleagues.

Alcoholism affects the entire family. An alcoholic is stuck in his problem. His whole family in their efforts and desire to help gets pulled down too. The family has to be solid and tough with its feet right on the ground if it wants to help. It's not a rare situation that parents split up if their child is an alcoholic. Alcohol can cause break down of the family.

Alcohol also affects the partner. It isn't easy to live with a person whose drinking causes problems. The drinker is full of conflicts, torn between alcohol and the need to drink and not wanting the harm anyone. Alcoholics often blame others when things are bad. The partner starts doubting, even questioning himself. He or she is trying to find a solution how to help the other partner, or how to protect children, or whether he or she should hide this from family, friends, and neighbors. The partner is often scared, ashamed or hurt.

The son or daughter of a parent who is an alcoholic can adopt different roles. He may be the one trying to help or go to the other side, start copying his parent. If, on the other hand, a child is an alcoholic, this can destroy the family. Parents start fighting, very often blaming each other.

Alcoholism can simply be described as a destroyer. It destroys the person who drinks and everyone connected with him. You've already seen how much it affects a family, a partner and children. We can't forget to tell that it also tears friendships apart.

From this short part of my book you can see that alcohol addiction affects everything and everyone. It's hard for everyone around the addicted person so, please, next time you get drunk, or tend to, think about people who love you and care about you. You don't just destroy your life, you destroy theirs, too.

Staying away from the first drink

When you take your first drink, you don't see how that can destroy your life. You never want more than one or two drinks. But, in time you increase the number. Then, later, as you grow older, you drink more and more.

If this bothers us, we control ourselves-we drink one, maybe two drinks. In this case we are very well aware of the consequences and we know our limits. But, it happens that instead of limiting we start hiding how much we drink. If you know how and can limit yourself, that's good. You'll have a drink from time to time, in special occasions and that's ok.

Sometimes people think they are experienced in drinking and no matter how much they drink they've got everything under control. Oh, but the experience is often a trap. Yes, you've heard me, a trap. That trap tells you that you can drink safely. And then- BUM. You are drunk again.

Then, how to stay away from that first drink? There is a saying that says "If you don't take your first drink, you don't get drunk". This is purely logical. The solution seems simply because it is. Instead of trying to limit yourself or planning not to get drunk avoid just one drink-the first one. End it before it had even started. Don't count how many drinks is ok, or how much you can drink before you pass out, just, simply,

don'   take   the   first   one.
Staying away from the first drink is a huge challenge, especially because the influence is big (alcohol is everywhere around us). If you feel challenged make yourselves busy, find an extra activity, read, start writing, finish college, go running, or call your mum. Do anything you like except drinking. If you persuade yourself to skip that first one you've already won.

The myth of the addictive personality

Do you agree with the opinion that life is a combination of addictions? Many of us will say that we are, in some way, addicted to coffee, or tea, maybe shopping, our work, or television. The real question is, can this be called addiction?

The first problem is how to define addiction. We use the words *addiction* or *addictive* so much in everyday life that, some would say, this word lost its meaning. The issue is what is the difference between a healthy enthusiasm and an addiction? We may say that the first is an addition to life while the other one is a taker. Addiction must comprise certain components (conflicts, preoccupation, disability, and increase in behavior, losing control, etc.). It might be useful to think of addictions as problems.

When we think of someone with an addictive personality, we usually imagine it looking bad, weak, selfish, unreliable, and out of control. The temper of these people is seen as defective, of bad influence.

But, don't you agree that this picture is maybe exaggerated? I would personally say yes, it is. This is more racial point of view than it's really the truth.

Psychiatrists tried to confirm the idea of addictive personality but, despite their efforts, they didn't find addictive personality common to everyone.

Not all people who have defective or selfish personality are addicted. To be honest, the idea of a general addictive personality is actually a myth. Psychiatrists and other researchers couldn't find universal characteristics common to all addicted people. Many of them can control their addiction while others can't. We are talking about completely different personalities and physical look. We have addicted people who are thin, or fat, bold, shy, bad, cruel, or kind and sensitive. There is no a stereotype.

Even though we cannot determine common characteristics for addicted people, there is a possibility to determine who is at high risk (this refers to both, people who are antisocial and knotty and those who are over sensitive). People who are impulsive and like trying out new things and adventures are at high risk. But, the number of addicted people who don't like new things or are compulsive is not negligible.

Many different factor influence the development of the addiction. Also, many different behavioral problems appear at certain age (especially among teenagers) with those who drink and those who don't (depression, anxiety, and delinquent behavior).

People who drink moderately (not nondrinkers) adjust best, at least there where drinking is some type of a social norm. Middle is the best, not extremes.

I would like to point out here that there is a possibility to see some specific details about whether the person can become addicted in advance, or better said on time. This means it's possible to predict addiction. It's common for those (especially males) who are impulsive, bold, adventurous to conceive some type of addiction. Among women, emotions like being often sad or anxious can be predictors. Of course this doesn't always mean that a person will become alcoholic. On one side, we've got adventurous personality and on the other, sad and anxious person. These two are not mutually exclusive .So the third factor or better to say indicator is the combination of the first two. This involves many contradictions in one person. On first sight, these three have nothing in common. But, if we look closer, all three have a thing in common-problems with self-regulation. And this problem is not a problem with a personality disorder.

To conclude, it's wrong to think that there is a disorder called addictive personality. You can't be born with it and there are no genes you could inherit to cause this. If you became addictive it's because you thought that it was the easiest solution of your problems and you should fight to win. If, on the other hand you want to help someone who is already addicted, don't find excuses for your loved ones in addicted personality.

Those lucky normal drinkers

Does this really exist? I'll try to answer this very common question although I'm not so sure that anyone can answer this precisely. Most alcoholics ask themselves very often if there is such a thing as a normal drinker. There is a difference between drinking a little and excessive drinking. I've mentioned earlier that the best way could be moderate drinking. Normal drinking refers to people who can drink and not drink at the same time. This means that they can take a drink or two in some occasions, but they don't need a drink all the time, in all the occasions. These "normal drinkers" can solve the problems without alcohol. But there are many people who spend their entire life drinking from time to time. How can they say they are not alcoholics? Well, they can't.

Thinking about addicted alcoholics as different species, is wrong. Those are just people who (from different reasons) found an easy way out of hard life, and problems, maybe loneliness and started drinking. If there is a difference between heavy drinking and normal drinking, I would say it is just in the amount of alcohol. For some people moderate drinking is normal, for other people it isn't. The best way is not to drink at all.

But, when we look around, we'll see that alcohol became a part of social life and sometimes it's simply inevitable. My advice to you, who start drinking, especially young people, is to clear your thoughts, think twice and learn how to control drinking. Once you cross the line, it will be hard to come back.

How to make it easy to quit

There are many reasons to stop drinking alcohol. Some people need to stop drinking because of their medical problems, or because they started taking medication which mustn't be combined with alcohol. Others do this for religious reasons, or simply want to lead a healthier lifestyle.

If you think you're having drinking problems, go talk to a professional, a doctor, or turn to some support group. You can ask them for advice, or make sure that you are really addicted. Giving up drinking may not be easy (especially for heavy drinkers). There are some rules you need to follow to achieve this.

Accepting that you have a problem is the first and the most important step. Next is telling family and friends that you want to stop drinking. This way you will not only show good will and share your success but also gain support you will definitely need to keep you on the right track.

In the beginning the best is to avoid temptations. You should avoid situations or places, even people who tempt you to drink. Complete the time you used for drinking with some other activities. If you, for example had a habit to go for a drink after a working day, instead to a bar, go to the cinema. Exercises are also great so, go swimming or running, or go practicing in a gym.

One more important step is to determine the "triggers"-situations that caused drinking. When you identify them you'll know what to avoid.

It's not easy to completely start drinking, especially if you are a heavy drinker. If you've already made a decision to stop and head to a healthy life, do it gradually. At first, cut down the amount of alcohol you consume. It's easier this way and it's a good way to completely stop drinking in the future. For example, if you drink every day or night, try skipping every second day or night.

Changes can be hard and you should reward yourself for every step you make. Don't be hard on yourself. Try replacing your drink with fresh juice or something else. Put money you've spent on drinks aside and use it for something else. Trust me you'll be proud of yourself. Set your goal and follow it. Enjoy the benefits (you'll be happier, healthier, capable of socializing, you'll sleep better, lose weight, etc.).

In the end, be prepared that there are alcohol withdrawal problems such as trembling, headache, sweating, lack of appetite and others. Don't be scared, it will pass. Talk to a professional and ask for advice and support. There are medications that your doctor can prescribe and that will help. It's not an easy path but it's worth all the trouble.

The final drink

It seems impossible. Well, it isn't. Hard-yes, impossible-no. Remember your first drink. When did it happen, who with, why? Go through the period you were drinking. How many situations did you forget? How many friends have you lost and how many terrible things you did and said? I bet you can't even remember. Imagine how many good parties you've missed. Most important, how many days or maybe years you threw away for nothing. How many lost chances?

So many questions, so much lost time, so many missed opportunities. And only one reason-alcohol. Incredible, don't you think? You gave up everything for alcohol. And you've gained what? Nothing, my dear, nothing, that's what. So now, imagine your future without alcohol. You won't miss parties. You won't lose friends. You will have memories. You won't miss opportunities. Future, that should be your reason. Fight for it. Admit, decide and go for it. There is nothing to lose-just alcohol. Once you admit you have a problem and think about what I wrote, you'll make a decision. The decision that life without alcohol can be hard but also great. You will cry but also laugh.

You will fall but get up. So, my dear, tonight when you take that glass of wine or beer or maybe scotch, put it on your desk, say to it that it is the last. Take a deep breath and grab your chance. Your new life is waiting for you. Smile.

Can't seem to quit drinking?

Know why…. Addiction cripples the mind and body. When it comes to alcohol, it becomes difficult to shun since it is easily available and socially accepted. There are also other reasons, which make quitting drinking a very difficult task. Some of them are:

Your System demands it

If you are addicted to alcohol, you would need a bottle at specific hours of the day. Your entire nervous system and sensory organs would keep on pushing you beyond control. This is what perhaps makes quitting drinking such an uphill task! Even if you are mentally tough enough, you can easily fail to ignore this constant demand for alcohol. You will thus need greater mental capacity to be in a position to say no to alcohol something that most addicts may lack since they have no control over the alcohol but rather the alcohol controls them.

Lack of will power

Most alcohol addicts, including you, are well aware of the bad effects it has, yet you prefer to continue. This is because most alcohol addicts do not have enough will power or determination to stay away from it. You have certainly tried avoiding it for a certain length of time; however, you have failed. You constantly end up finding some sort of excuse for that iconic "one last drink", which never is.

Lack of Counseling

When it comes to quitting alcohol, it is 70% a mind job and 30% physical job. Most of the addicts are not mentally tough enough to continue their battle against alcohol for a long time; they eventually end up filling their glass. Proper counseling can help here. A good counselor can help an individual gain that level of self-confidence and determination, which is a prime requisite to giving up drinking.

Unless you make up your mind to quit drinking for a better life then I can confidently tell you that you will never quit drinking. No magic program or magic pill will help you stop drinking; the first thing you need to do is to come out of denial, accept that you have a problem and be willing to change your life for the better. Just saying that you will drink over the weekends and holidays only will not just cut it. Trust me, it just takes one drink and another drink and before you know it, you have had too many and you are back to your drinking.

13 Amazing Reasons to Stop Drinking

These 13 interesting reasons are going to motivate you to stop intake of alcohol and become sober within no time.

*You will sleep soundly with almost inaudible snoring. Yeah...your spouse is going to rejoice.

*You will smell original and will leave behind the brewery-odor you always used to carry with you.

*Your bloated paunch is going to subside now, making you look smarter than ever before.

*You will look beyond alcohol towards so many beautiful things. Your family will enjoy with you without any fear of you getting bananas after a couple of drinks.

*You can go anywhere you want and do whatever you like without worrying about your drinking schedule that you hated to disrupt earlier.

*You will rediscover the taste and health of refreshing fruit and vegetable juices.

*Time will suddenly seem to have slowed down for you. You will now have abundant of time at your disposal.

*You will start distinguishing good TV shows from bad ones simply because you watched every show that ran on TV oblivious to what it was showing. What used to enthrall you earlier will seem too absurd now.

*You will become more observant and will explore your creative self, something you were never aware about.

*You will realize your work productivity has increased. Earlier, you were as lazy as an ass. Who knows, you could get that promotion that you had always been desiring.

*Your mornings are going to become really special. There is going to be zero hangovers and headaches unlike earlier 'drunk mornings'.

*How beautiful the sunrise is going to appear to you!

*You will handle your emotions much better and address problems head on rather than turning to alcohol to numb your senses.

Start With 15-Days Of Sobriety

Take One Day At A Time

Now, since you have come out of denial and looking forward to look and feel good without alcohol, start with this 15-day schedule of sobriety. This is going to be commencement of your de-addiction. Take life as it comes each day and do not think beyond that day. Read these messages for the next 15 days for knocking that bottle off from your life. If you happen to discontinue this 15-days routine, pick up from where you left.

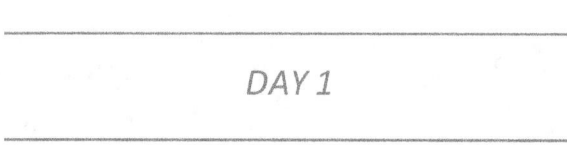

DAY 1

Say to self - "To make the changes I want, I need to let go of unhealthy stuff" Today will mark the beginning of your abstinence. Take each situation one step at a time. Every time you feel pressure, you are closer to success. Be proud of each success and reward yourself at the end of the day.

DAY 2

Say to self - "Promises materialize if we work for them". Plan your time to evade boredom. Buy a magazine or book. Take a 10 minute walk. Drink lots of water. Every time urges hit, eat an apple or two. This is the second day of your success so don't forget to reward yourself.

DAY 3

Say to self - "Let faith be alive in me round the clock!" Get rid of all alcohol bottles, beer cans, glasses etc. Buy something for yourself. Work out today to feel better about this decision.

DAY 4

Say to self - "Live in the world of only now with no shadows of yesterdays or clouds of tomorrow". Find something to do with your hands like playing an instrument. Keep yourself hydrated. Plan an activity with your siblings.

DAY 5

Say to self -"I congratulate myself" Remind yourself about how you have revived your health and started to improve. Stay motivated and feel great. Breathe deeply and get yourself inspired.

DAY 6

Say to self - "I am in control of my life". Calculate how much money you have saved in the last 5 days. The total can be several hundreds of dollars. Pat yourself on the back for the work well done so far. Begin saving for holidays, shopping, or may be your favorite concert.

DAY 7

Say to self - "I will be attentive to nutrition". Concentrate on filling your body nutritious foods. Beware of the extra calories and find more time to work out. Replace the calories with nutritious foods. Consume fresh fruit, fresh vegetables, vegetable juices, skimmed milk, and plain yogurt.

DAY 8

Say to self – "I am part way through the battle!" You have successfully led an alcohol free weekend. You will now take it week by week and even longer. Have the right attitude and identify benefits of this change. Promise not to give in to an urge.

DAY 9

Say to self – "I will think positively". Some of the strongest cravings come with specific people, events or places. Divert your mind with the help of music or some sport. Sing loudly and yes, like you are crazy! Nibble toothpick while driving. Try not to be in company of drinking friends. Stay away from them.

Say to self – "I am full of strength" Imagine a changed you. Revere the valuable people in your life and how they inspire you. Start working on a new image and start achieving goals from the list you made. Whenever someone offers you a drink, say out loud, 'No thanks'.

Say to self – "My breath is my life". Do an exercise where there is use of deep breathing for the relaxing and euphoric effect. Let yourself relax by going limp. Inhale deeply and slowly. Practice this exercise few times every day.

DAY 12

Say to self – "Everything is possible." Promise yourself not to have a drink. Congratulate yourself on the progress made so far. Remember that you are committed to yourself.

DAY 13

Say to self – "I am master of my choices" Identify all the traps that may be surrounding you. Don't fall for them. One common and discreet trap is overconfidence that may make you feel alcohol is not a big deal for you. You might think that you can handle one or two bottles. I assure you that you cannot so don't even go there. Another probable trap could be crises that come with a feeling of pain or guilt propelling you towards alcohol intake. Remain prepared to handle these traps.

DAY 14

Say to self – "I won't resort to excuses". You may take a step, or may be two, backward while moving ahead on the track of alcohol abstinence. This is normal and must be taken in stride. It is important to not stop and keep on scaling pointers.

DAY 15

Say to self – "Congratulations. I am proud of myself". Realize that you have been without alcohol for a fortnight. This is a positive onset of your liberation. Use all the time you have lost in enjoying things around you. Take life a day at a time and focus on its positivity. Celebrate by doing something good for yourself! Remember that in the first days, you will experience some withdrawal symptoms like insomnia, excessive sweating, anxiety, high blood pressure and indigestion. You will need to know how to deal with them if you are to be successful. A support network is very important in ensuring that you remain on track as well as provide the appropriate guidance in your journey for sobriety.

What If I Trip?

Your journey to gain sobriety will not be easy. But don't get bogged down. If you happen to fall into the trap, these tips will be of great help— Halt – If you have become drunk even after abstaining for a consistent period, just stop again. Don't give in to this slip. Just STOP at once. Acknowledge the slip – Yeah...you are feeling guilty after the slip. It is good to be guilty as it shows you are changing and want to continue the process. Let go of your disappointment and guilt to start again. Stay honest – Do not fool yourself by evading the slip and its consequences. Get active in knowing what made you succumb and how it can be prevented. Gather the help you may need and start afresh. Seek help – It's good that you want to tackle your alcoholism self-reliantly, but seek help from your loved ones for better and quicker results. Ponder what made you trip – Acknowledge the causes of pitfalls and work towards them. Make your approach goal-oriented. Cut off – Regain the control and cut off all the chances to trip again. Take good care of your body and mind. Remember: *Intoxication is not synonymous with pleasure *Your drinking buddies will always encourage you to drink. *There is nothing called sustainable happiness happiness that comes from drinking. *Hang around with healthy and sober friends. *Weigh your decisions and emotions judiciously.

Here is how you are going to feel day by day as you shun alcohol: In few days your skin will look hydrated again after suffering sapping of its moisture by your alcoholic drinks. It will start looking good and shiny. The capillaries that have been swollen for such a long time will retain normalcy and make your skin look relatively good. Your liver will fall in love with you for giving it a fresh bout of life. It will work better and faster. Suddenly you will find your bruises, burns and cuts recovering rapidly. The acid reflux will start subsiding and digestion will be superb. In a week or two your mind will become clearer and fog of depression will subside. Your family will get to see you in a better mood. By this time, your heart will also fall in love with you since it has to work lighter now. Your pulse rate will normalize and your body will start getting back within your control. In a month's time your bloated belly is getting normal now. Your abs are going to make a sensational comeback and your friends are going to be jealous of you. Your body and your mind are resting better, as you sleep soundly now You can work longer and add to your professional productivity. Even your partner is going to notice the change in your libido.

Dealing With Guilt

We have all experienced guilt at some point in our lives, but perhaps us addicts are guilty of (no pun intended) feeling this emotion the most.

Generally speaking, guilt is an emotion that can serve us well, ensuring that we learn from our past mistakes, or to warn us that something we have or haven't done isn't quite right. We can feel this emotion on a powerful level, but sometimes it can simply remain in the background like a dull cloud of unease.

I have found that, from an addict's perspective, there are two types of guilt: the kind of guilt that leads to addiction, and the kind that is caused by it.

Guilt that leads to addiction doesn't technically have anything to do with addiction itself. It can be categorised as a sense of hopelessness or regret caused because you feel that you have done or not done something that could cause someone or something to suffer. That "so meone" could be you, your partner, your children, your friends, your colleagues or a complete stranger. The "s omething" could be your job, your home, your possessions, your money, your pets, the government, the state of the world and any other thing over which you can justify feeling guilty.

In reality, you may or may not have been a factor in your perceived suffering of this person or thing. In either case, it doesn't matter because you already feel bad for letting down this person or thing. This is dangerous territory for an addict, because it can generate self hate or self pity, either of which can be used as justification to indulge in your addiction.

Guilt that is caused by addiction - you feel bad for giving in to your addiction, you lied to cover it up, wasted money, stole, etc - is a clear sign that you are currently at odds with your addiction. On the other hand, addiction guilt can be used as an ally. For starters, the fact that you feel guilty is a positive sign - it means you feel remorse over your actions and don't want or intend to cause harm to anyone. It also means you recognise that things need to change.

In any case, guilt is always either about what you did or didn't do. This means you have two options: either accept things for what they are and forgive yourself, or take action now to rectify the situation. If you decide not to follow either of these options, then it's likely that you will continue feeling guilty indefinitely.

Only you have the power to stop feeling guilty, whether you choose to weather the storm and learn to forgive yourself, or you come clean and make amends. Neither option is the right nor wrong one - whichever of these most resonates with you and seems most fitting to your personal circumstances should be considered.

The past is always the past. It's gone, dead, now just a memory leaving only now and a future yet to be written. Everything you have ever thought of and acted upon in the past has lead you to now. So, now is the time to move forward without looking back. And whenever that niggling voice in your head says "you can't move on, haven't you forgotten what you did?", simply push it away. In the words of Dr. Evil, simply tell all such mental chatter to "zip it!" All self-effacing chatter is just habitual. The fact is, you want to better yourself - so you must discard the old baggage in order to embrace the present and feel hopeful of the future.

I want you to do something now. If you are currently in or regularly find yourself in a state of guilt, I want you to re-read the above paragraph - several times. Push the guilty mental chatter away whenever it begins to appear. If you catch your mind dwelling on this guilt, then push the thought away with a quick, sharp inhalation of breath and re-read the above paragraph.

Life After Addiction

The saying "once an addict, always an addict" holds an element of truth. After all, addiction has a highly emotive charge to it and the memories of this difficult and potentially traumatic time in your life may stay with you for a long time following successful recovery.

Don't get me wrong - life as a recovering addict gets far easier with time. The more you experience life free from the shackles of addiction, the more first-hand experience you have of actually knowing that you are better off without it. This prompts you to daydream increasingly less on your addiction, reducing the chances of an addictive pull from arising. And, as we've learnt, beating addiction without a physical pull present is far easier. You'll begin thinking less about your addictive past, you'll give very little thought to any wrongs you may have committed as a result of your dependencies - dwelling on such matters serves nobody; it's time to move on. And the sooner you move on, the sooner you'll forget entirely that you were ever addicted to something at all. What was once a major part of your life and which comprised a huge percentage of your daily thoughts now becomes but a distant memory, like a fragmented bundle of thoughts from another time, of another person. As with all memories of difficult times, even these soon dissolve into obscurity, dreamlike, just a wisp of an emotion. The memory can be accessed but the emotional baggage of it has either disappeared entirely or is now so insignificant that it barely shows up on your radar, so to speak.

Curiously, over time you may still occasionally experience a form of physical pull, particularly during upsetting or difficult periods in your life. But by this time you will have dissociated entirely from your addiction. These pulls are therefore just physical symptoms of an underlying emotion. Your addiction has ended, it's a thing of the past, therefore you now employ your strong will to successfully ignore the physical symptoms and you simply get on with your life, free from any crutches or dependencies. You may even smile inwardly when the pull arises - an old enemy now seems weak, powerless - because in hindsight the pull was never really the issue; it was your lack of will.

Yes, the pull was most likely in the background all along, even before you were an addict. I believe that all of us - addicts or otherwise - all suffer with this pull, this yearning for more, for a solution to our human dilemma. Some of us simply turn to addictive behaviour, compulsive dependencies, as a shortcut or a way of making sense of this apparent need for more. But now you have the power to live life without this dependency. Now you have truly found your free will. This is what life as a recovering addict is like. Are you ready?

information is without contract or any type of guarantee assurance.

The trademarks that are used are without any consent, and the publication of the trademark is without permission or backing by the trademark owner. All trademarks and brands within this book are for clarifying purposes only and are the owned by the owners themselves, not affiliated with this document.